The Radiant Force

Harnessing The Power of Positivity

Mark Winters

The Radiant Force: Harnessing The Power of Positivity

Author Mark Winters

Published By Neil McKenzie

ISBN 9781445217154
Imprint: Lulu.com

In a world often overshadowed by negativity, the journey towards a positive mindset can seem like an elusive quest. However, within every individual lies the potential to cultivate positivity, transforming lives and shaping destinies. "The Radiant Force" delves into the profound impact of positivity, illuminating its transformative power and providing practical insights to unleash its radiance in every aspect of life.

Chapter 1:

Understanding Positivity

- Defining Positivity:

Exploring the Essence of Positivity and its Multifaceted Manifestations.

- The Science Behind Positivity:

Unveiling the Neurological and Psychological Underpinnings of Positive Thinking.

- The Ripple Effect:

Examining How positivity Influences Personal Well-being, Relationships, and Societal Dynamics.

Chapter 2:

Overcoming Negativity Bias

- Recognising Negativity Bias:

Understanding the Innate Tendency to Dwell on Negative Experiences.

- Flipping the Script:

Techniques to Reframe Negative Thoughts and Cultivate an Optimistic Outlook.

- Embracing Resilience:

Nurturing the Ability to Bounce Back from Setbacks and Adversities.

Chapter 3:

Cultivating a Positive Mindset

- Gratitude and Appreciation:

Embracing Gratitude as a Gateway to Positivity and Fulfilment.

Mindfulness and Presence:

Practices to Anchor Oneself in the Present Moment and Savour Life's Joys.

Self-Compassion:

Fostering Kindness and Acceptance Towards Oneself Amidst Life's Challenges

Chapter 4:

Empowering Relationships

- The Power of Connection:

Exploring How Positive Relationships
Enrich Our Lives and Nurture Our Well-
being.

- Communicating with Positivity:

Techniques for fostering constructive
communication and resolving conflicts.

- Building Support Networks:

Cultivating Relationships That Uplift,
Inspire, and Sustain Us Through Life's
Trials.

Chapter 5:

Pursuing Purpose and Meaning

- Aligning with Values:

Discovering and Living in Alignment with Personal Values and Aspirations.

- Finding Flow:

Engaging in Activities That Foster Immersion, Creativity, and a Sense of Purpose.

- Contribution and Service:

Harnessing the Transformative Power of Giving Back to Others and Making a Difference in the World.

Chapter 6:

Navigating Challenges with Optimism

- Resilient Optimism:

Cultivating a Resilient Mindset That Sees Setbacks as Opportunities for Growth.

- Adaptive Coping Strategies:

Techniques for Navigating Challenges with Grace, Creativity, and Resilience.

- The Role of Perspective:

Harnessing the Power of Perspective to Find Meaning and Wisdom in Life's Trials.

Chapter 7:

Sustaining Positivity Amidst Adversity

- Weathering Storms:

Strategies for Maintaining Positivity During Times of Crisis, Uncertainty, and Grief.

- The Role of Self-Care:

Prioritizing Self-care Practices that Nourish the Mind, Body, and Spirit.

- Seeking Support:

Leveraging the Support of Others and seeking Professional Help when Needed.

Embracing Positivity:

 A Call to Radiate Transformative Energy into the World

Chapter 1:

Understanding Positivity

- Defining Positivity:

Exploring the Essence of Positivity and its Multifaceted Manifestations.

- The Science Behind Positivity:

Unveiling the Neurological and Psychological Underpinnings of Positive Thinking.

Understanding Positivity

In the vast tapestry of human experience, the power of positivity weaves a thread that illuminates the darkest corners of our minds and hearts. It is not merely a fleeting emotion but a profound mindset that shapes our perceptions, influences our actions, and ultimately determines the quality of our lives. Understanding positivity transcends the superficiality of mere optimism; it delves deep into the core of our being, fostering resilience, empathy, and a profound sense of interconnectedness.

At its essence, positivity is not the denial of life's challenges or the dismissal of pain and suffering. Instead, it is the conscious choice to perceive difficulties as opportunities for growth, setbacks as lessons in resilience, and moments of despair as catalysts for profound transformation. It is a mindset that acknowledges the complexities of existence yet refuses to be shackled by negativity.

To truly understand positivity is to embrace the inherent duality of the human experience—the light and the shadow, the joy and the sorrow. It is to recognize that within every adversity lies the seed of opportunity, waiting to be nurtured by the fertile soil of our resilience and determination.

Cultivating a mindset of positivity requires a willingness to engage in self-reflection and introspection. It involves reframing our perspectives, challenging limiting beliefs, and practicing gratitude for the abundance that surrounds us, no matter how obscured it may seem in moments of darkness.

Moreover, understanding positivity entails extending compassion and empathy not only to ourselves but also to others. It is recognizing that we are all interconnected, that our actions and words have the power to uplift or diminish those around us. By fostering a sense of unity and interconnectedness, we not only enrich our own lives but also contribute to the collective well-being of humanity.

In the journey toward understanding positivity, resilience emerges as a guiding principle—a steadfast anchor that grounds us amidst life's tumultuous seas. Resilience is not the absence of adversity but the ability to bounce back from setbacks with newfound strength and wisdom. It is a testament to the human spirit's capacity for growth and transformation, a beacon of hope that illuminates even the darkest of nights.

Ultimately, embracing positivity is a choice—a choice to see the beauty in the world, to find meaning in the mundane, and to approach life with an open heart and mind. It is a commitment to living authentically, with intention and purpose, and to inspiring others to do the same.

Understanding positivity transcends mere optimism; it is a profound mindset that shapes our perceptions, influences our actions, and enriches our lives. By embracing resilience, fostering empathy, and cultivating gratitude, we can harness the transformative power of positivity to create a brighter, more compassionate world for ourselves and future generations.

Defining Positivity:

Exploring the essence of positivity and its multifaceted manifestations.

Positivity, like a multifaceted gem, sparkles with brilliance and depth, revealing different facets depending on how the light of perception strikes it. It is a force that permeates every aspect of our lives, shaping our thoughts, emotions, and actions in profound ways. Yet, defining positivity proves to be as elusive as grasping the shifting hues of a kaleidoscope, for its essence transcends simple categorization or reduction.

At its core, positivity embodies a mindset of hope, resilience, and gratitude—a lens through which we perceive the world with openness and optimism. It is the unwavering belief in the inherent goodness of life, despite its inevitable challenges and uncertainties. Positivity is not a mere state of mind but a way of being —an orientation towards life that fosters growth, connection, and well-being.

One of the most recognizable manifestations of positivity is optimism—the hopeful outlook that sees possibilities where others see obstacles, and opportunities where others see limitations. Optimism empowers us to face adversity with courage and determination, knowing that every setback is but a stepping stone on the path to success.

Yet, positivity extends far beyond the realm of optimism, encompassing a myriad of other qualities and attitudes that enrich our lives and uplift our spirits. Gratitude, for instance, is a potent expression of positivity—a humble acknowledgment of the blessings, both big and small, that grace our lives each day. By cultivating gratitude, we cultivate a deep sense of appreciation for the richness of existence, finding joy in the simplest of moments and treasures in the mundane.

Similarly, resilience emerges as a hallmark of positivity —an indomitable spirit that rises from the ashes of adversity, stronger and more resilient than before. Resilience is not the absence of hardship but the ability to adapt, grow, and thrive in the face of challenges, drawing strength from the depths of our inner resources.

Compassion, too, lies at the heart of positivity—a boundless wellspring of kindness, empathy, and understanding that transcends barriers of culture, creed, and circumstance. It is through compassion that we forge meaningful connections with others, fostering a sense of unity and solidarity that transcends the boundaries of self.

Moreover, positivity finds expression not only in our relationships with others but also in our relationship with ourselves. Self-love, self-compassion, and self-care are essential pillars of positivity, nurturing our inner well-being and fostering a deep sense of inner peace and contentment.

In essence, defining positivity is akin to capturing the essence of life itself—a dynamic interplay of light and shadow, joy and sorrow, growth and transformation. It is a journey of exploration and discovery—a quest to uncover the hidden depths of our own hearts and minds and to embrace the boundless potential that lies within.

As we navigate the twists and turns of life's journey, may we cultivate the essence of positivity in all its multifaceted manifestations, embracing optimism, gratitude, resilience, and compassion with open hearts and minds. For in the radiant glow of positivity, we find the courage to dream, the strength to persevere, and the wisdom to embrace life's infinite possibilities.

The Science Behind Positivity:

Unveiling the neurological and psychological underpinnings of positive thinking.

In the intricate landscape of the human mind, the phenomenon of positive thinking emerges as a beacon of hope, resilience, and well-being. Yet, beneath its surface lies a complex interplay of neurological and psychological mechanisms that shape our perceptions, emotions, and behaviours. Delving into the science behind positivity unveils a fascinating tapestry of neural pathways, neurotransmitters, and cognitive processes that illuminate the transformative power of a positive mindset.

At the neurological level, positive thinking is intricately linked to the functioning of the brain's reward system—a network of neural circuits that respond to pleasurable stimuli and reinforce adaptive behaviours. Key structures within this system include the nucleus accumbens, the ventral tegmental area, and the prefrontal cortex, which work in concert to regulate mood, motivation, and decision-making.

When we experience moments of joy, gratitude, or contentment, the brain releases a cascade of neurotransmitters, including dopamine, serotonin, and endorphins, which flood the reward pathways, creating a sense of pleasure and well-being. These neurochemicals not only enhance mood but also promote resilience, cognitive flexibility, and social bonding, laying the foundation for a positive outlook on life.

Moreover, neuroplasticity—the brain's remarkable ability to reorganize and adapt in response to experience—plays a crucial role in shaping our capacity for positive thinking. Through repeated engagement in positive thoughts and behaviours, we strengthen neural connections associated with optimism, resilience, and emotional regulation, effectively rewiring the brain to perceive the world through a more hopeful and optimistic lens.

From a psychological perspective, positive thinking is closely intertwined with cognitive processes such as attention, interpretation, and memory. The renowned psychologist Barbara Fredrickson proposed the "broaden-and-build" theory, which suggests that positive emotions broaden our awareness and cognitive resources, enabling us to approach life with curiosity, creativity, and openness.

By expanding our cognitive repertoire, positive emotions facilitate flexible thinking and problem-solving, allowing us to generate novel solutions and adapt to changing circumstances more effectively. Furthermore, positivity bias—the tendency to focus on and remember positive information more readily than negative information— serves as a protective mechanism that shields us from the detrimental effects of stress and adversity.

Through the practice of mindfulness and meditation, we can cultivate greater awareness and acceptance of our thoughts and emotions, fostering a deeper sense of presence and inner peace. These practices have been shown to modulate activity in brain regions associated with emotion regulation, attention, and self-awareness, promoting a more balanced and resilient mindset.

In conclusion, the science behind positivity offers a compelling insight into the intricate interplay of neurological and psychological processes that underlie our capacity for positive thinking. By understanding the neural mechanisms and cognitive pathways through which positivity operates, we can harness its transformative power to cultivate resilience, enhance well-being, and enrich our lives. As we continue to unravel the mysteries of the human mind, may we embrace the science of positivity as a guiding light on the journey toward greater happiness, fulfilment, and flourishing.

The Ripple Effect:

Examining how positivity influences personal well-being, relationships, and societal dynamics

In the vast ocean of human interaction, every thought, word, and action create ripples that reverberate far beyond our immediate sphere of influence. At the heart of this intricate web of interconnectedness lies the transformative power of positivity—a force that transcends individual boundaries and shapes the fabric of our collective experience. By examining the ripple effect of positivity, we uncover its profound influence on personal well-being, relationships, and the dynamics of society at large.

Personal Well-being:

Positivity serves as a catalyst for personal growth and flourishing, nurturing a sense of inner peace, resilience, and fulfilment. Scientific research reveals that cultivating a positive mindset triggers a cascade of neurological and physiological responses in the brain and body. Positivity stimulates the release of neurotransmitters such as dopamine and endorphins, which are associated with feelings of happiness and well-being. Moreover, positive thinking has been linked to improved cardiovascular health, strengthened immune function, and enhanced overall resilience in the face of adversity.

Furthermore, individuals who embrace positivity are more likely to engage in healthy lifestyle behaviours, such as regular exercise, nutritious eating habits, and adequate sleep. By prioritizing self-care and emotional well-being, they create a foundation of resilience that enables them to navigate life's challenges with grace and optimism.

Relationships:

The ripple effect of positivity extends far beyond the confines of individual well-being, permeating the dynamics of interpersonal relationships. Positivity serves as a magnet for connection, fostering empathy, trust, and mutual support among friends, family members, and romantic partners.

Studies have shown that positive communication patterns, characterized by expressions of appreciation, encouragement, and affection, are key predictors of relationship satisfaction and longevity. Couples who cultivate a culture of positivity in their interactions are better equipped to weather conflicts and navigate disagreements constructively, strengthening the bonds of love and intimacy.

Moreover, the ripple effect of positivity extends beyond dyadic relationships to encompass broader social networks and communities. Acts of kindness, generosity, and compassion create a ripple effect that spreads outward, inspiring others to pay it forward and fostering a culture of altruism and collective well-being.

Societal Dynamics:

At the macroscopic level, the ripple effect of positivity exerts a transformative influence on the fabric of society, shaping cultural norms, institutions, and collective behaviours. Societies that prioritize values such as empathy, inclusivity, and social justice are more likely to cultivate environments that foster individual flourishing and collective prosperity.

Research suggests that positive social norms and collective beliefs can drive societal change by influencing the attitudes and behaviours of individuals within a community. For example, campaigns promoting environmental sustainability or public health initiatives rely on the power of positivity to mobilize collective action and inspire widespread participation.

Furthermore, the ripple effect of positivity can serve as a counterbalance to negative forces such as fear, prejudice, and division, fostering resilience and unity in the face of adversity. By amplifying voices of hope, resilience, and progress, societies can cultivate a shared sense of purpose and belonging that transcends cultural, ideological, and geographic boundaries.

In conclusion, the ripple effect of positivity extends its luminous tendrils into every facet of human experience, shaping the trajectory of individual lives, the dynamics of interpersonal relationships, and the evolution of society as a whole. By embracing positivity as a guiding principle, we harness its transformative power to create a world where well-being, connection, and collective flourishing are the currency of human interaction.

Chapter 2:

Overcoming Negativity Bias

- Recognizing Negativity Bias:

Understanding the Innate Tendency to Dwell on Negative Experiences.

- Flipping the Script:

Techniques to Reframe Negative Thoughts and Cultivate an Optimistic Outlook.

- Embracing Resilience:

Nurturing the Ability to Bounce Back from Setbacks and Adversities.

Overcoming Negative Bias

In the labyrinth of the human mind, negative bias lurks like a shadow, casting doubt and despair over our perceptions of the world. It is a cognitive phenomenon that predisposes us to focus on the negative aspects of life while overlooking the positive—a deeply ingrained survival mechanism shaped by evolutionary forces. However, by understanding the roots of negative bias and employing strategies to overcome it, we can unlock the door to a brighter, more optimistic outlook on life.

Negative bias stems from our brain's evolutionary wiring, which evolved to prioritize threats and dangers in order to ensure survival. In ancient times, this cognitive bias served a crucial purpose, alerting our ancestors to potential risks and enabling them to take swift action to protect themselves. However, in the modern world, where physical threats are less prevalent but psychological stressors abound, negative bias can become a hindrance rather than a help.

One of the key features of negative bias is its tendency to magnify negative experiences and downplay positive ones—a phenomenon known as negativity bias. This inherent tendency can lead us to dwell on setbacks, failures, and disappointments while discounting or overlooking moments of joy, success, and progress. As a result, our perceptions become skewed, and our overall outlook becomes disproportionately pessimistic.

Overcoming negative bias requires a conscious effort to retrain our brains and recalibrate our perceptions of the world. One powerful strategy is cognitive restructuring, which involves identifying and challenging negative thought patterns and replacing them with more balanced and realistic ones. By practicing mindfulness and self-awareness, we can learn to observe our thoughts without judgment and consciously choose to focus on the positive aspects of our experiences.

Cultivating gratitude is another effective antidote to negative bias, as it shifts our attention away from what is lacking or wrong and redirects it toward what we have to be thankful for. Keeping a gratitude journal, where we regularly jot down moments of appreciation and blessings, can help rewire our brains to recognize and savour the abundance in our lives.

Moreover, fostering a growth mindset—a belief that our abilities and intelligence are not fixed but can be developed through effort and perseverance—can counteract the tendency to view setbacks as insurmountable obstacles. By reframing failures as opportunities for learning and growth, we can cultivate resilience and optimism in the face of adversity.

Social support and positive relationships also play a crucial role in overcoming negative bias. Surrounding ourselves with supportive and uplifting individuals who share our values and aspirations can provide a buffer against the negative influences of the world. By nurturing meaningful connections and seeking out sources of inspiration and encouragement, we can create an environment that nurtures positivity and resilience.

In conclusion, overcoming negative bias is a journey of self-discovery and self-mastery—a process of rewiring our brains and transforming our perceptions of the world. By challenging negative thought patterns, cultivating gratitude, fostering a growth mindset, and nurturing positive relationships, we can break free from the shackles of pessimism and embrace a brighter, more hopeful outlook on life. In doing so, we not only enhance our own well-being but also contribute to the collective upliftment of humanity.

Recognising Negativity Bias:

Understanding the Innate Tendency to Dwell on Negative Experiences

In the labyrinth of the human mind, a subtle but powerful force shapes our perceptions, colouring the lens through which we view the world. This force, known as negativity bias, is a deeply ingrained cognitive phenomenon that predisposes us to focus on the negative aspects of life while downplaying the positive. By recognizing negativity bias and understanding its origins, we can begin to navigate its influence and cultivate a more balanced perspective on our experiences.

Negativity bias is rooted in our brain's evolutionary history, shaped by millennia of adaptation to an environment where survival often hinged on the ability to detect and respond to potential threats. In ancestral times, vigilance towards danger was essential for survival, leading our ancestors to prioritize negative stimuli as a means of self-preservation. This bias served as a survival advantage, allowing early humans to anticipate and avoid potential risks, such as predators, hostile environments, or scarce resources.

However, while negativity bias may have conferred an evolutionary advantage in the past, in the modern world, where physical threats are less prevalent but psychological stressors abound, it can become a hindrance to our well-being. Our brains are wired to react more strongly to negative stimuli than to positive ones, a phenomenon known as the negativity bias effect. This predisposition causes us to dwell on negative experiences, thoughts, and emotions, even when positive ones may outnumber them.

Understanding the innate tendency to dwell on negative experiences begins with recognizing the pervasive influence of negativity bias in our lives. From the mundane to the extraordinary, our perceptions are shaped by this cognitive filter, subtly colouring our interactions, decisions, and interpretations of the world around us. Whether it's fixating on a minor criticism amidst a sea of compliments or ruminating over past failures while overlooking successes, negativity bias exerts a powerful influence on our thoughts and behaviours.

Moreover, negativity bias is compounded by factors such as social comparison, media exposure, and cultural conditioning, which reinforce and perpetuate our predisposition towards negativity. Social media platforms, in particular, can exacerbate negativity bias by amplifying sensationalist content and fostering a culture of comparison and envy. As a result, we may find ourselves constantly comparing our lives to others' highlight reels, leading to feelings of inadequacy, insecurity, and discontent.

However, while negativity bias may be a natural and instinctive tendency, it is not immutable. By cultivating awareness and mindfulness, we can begin to recognize when negativity bias is at play in our lives and consciously choose to shift our focus towards more positive and empowering perspectives. Practices such as mindfulness meditation, cognitive reframing, and gratitude journaling can help interrupt negative thought patterns and rewire our brains to adopt a more balanced and optimistic outlook.

Furthermore, fostering self-compassion and acceptance can help mitigate the impact of negativity bias by allowing us to acknowledge and validate our emotions without judgment or self-criticism. By embracing our inherent humanity, with all its imperfections and vulnerabilities, we can cultivate greater resilience and self-compassion in the face of life's inevitable challenges.

In conclusion, recognizing negativity bias and understanding its innate tendency to dwell on negative experiences is the first step towards transcending its influence and cultivating a more balanced and resilient mindset. By cultivating awareness, practicing mindfulness, and fostering self-compassion, we can begin to navigate the labyrinth of our minds with greater clarity, wisdom, and equanimity, ultimately reclaiming agency over our thoughts and perceptions.

Flipping the Script:

Techniques to Reframe Negative Thoughts and Cultivate an Optimistic Outlook

In the narrative of our lives, the stories we tell ourselves shape our perceptions, beliefs, and ultimately, our reality. Yet, amidst the ebb and flow of daily existence, negative thoughts often weave themselves into the fabric of our inner dialogue, casting shadows over our hopes and aspirations. Flipping the script entails rewriting these narratives, transforming pessimism into optimism and cultivating a mindset imbued with resilience, hope, and possibility. Here are several techniques to help reframe negative thoughts and nurture an optimistic outlook:

1. Identify Negative Thought Patterns:

The first step in flipping the script is to become aware of negative thought patterns as they arise. Pay attention to recurring themes or triggers that evoke feelings of self-doubt, fear, or despair. Journaling or mindfulness meditation can be invaluable tools for observing and documenting these thought patterns without judgment.

2. Challenge Negative Beliefs:

Once you have identified negative thought patterns, challenge the underlying beliefs that fuel them. Ask yourself: Is this thought based on factual evidence, or is it distorted by cognitive biases such as catastrophizing, black-and-white thinking, or mind reading? Examine the evidence objectively and consider alternative interpretations that are more balanced and realistic.

3. Practice Cognitive Reframing:

Cognitive reframing involves consciously changing the way you interpret and perceive situations to create a more positive narrative. When faced with a negative thought, reframe it by focusing on the silver lining or considering alternative perspectives. For example, instead of dwelling on a setback as a failure, view it as an opportunity for growth and learning.

4. Cultivate Gratitude:

Gratitude is a powerful antidote to negativity, shifting your focus from what is lacking to what is abundant in your life. Take time each day to reflect on the things you are grateful for, no matter how small or seemingly insignificant. Keeping a gratitude journal or practicing gratitude meditation can help cultivate a mindset of appreciation and abundance.

5. Set Realistic Goals: Unrealistic expectations can fuel feelings of disappointment and disillusionment when things don't go as planned. Set realistic, achievable goals that align with your values and priorities, and celebrate progress along the way. Break larger goals into smaller, manageable steps, and focus on the process rather than fixating solely on the outcome.

6. Practice Self-Compassion: Be kind and compassionate towards yourself, especially during challenging times. Treat yourself with the same level of understanding and empathy that you would offer to a friend facing similar circumstances. Practice self-care activities that nourish

your body, mind, and soul, whether it's taking a bubble bath, going for a nature walk, or indulging in a hobby you enjoy.

7. Surround Yourself with Positivity: Surround yourself with people, environments, and influences that uplift and inspire you. Seek out supportive friends and mentors who encourage your growth and celebrate your successes. Limit exposure to negative news or social media content that contributes to feelings of anxiety or despair, and instead, focus on sources of inspiration and positivity.

8. Practice Mindfulness: Mindfulness meditation can help cultivate awareness of your thoughts and emotions without getting caught up in them. Practice mindfulness techniques such as deep breathing, body scans, or mindful walking to anchor yourself in the present moment and cultivate a sense of calm and equanimity amidst life's ups and downs.

In conclusion, flipping the script involves consciously challenging negative thought patterns and cultivating a mindset of optimism, resilience, and possibility. By practicing cognitive reframing, cultivating gratitude, setting realistic goals, practicing self-compassion, surrounding yourself with positivity, and embracing mindfulness, you can rewrite the narratives that shape your perception of yourself and the world around you. As you embark on this journey of self-discovery and transformation, may you find the courage and strength to embrace the inherent potential for growth and fulfilment that resides within you.

Embracing Resilience:

Nurturing The Ability to Bounce Back from Setbacks and Adversities

In the tapestry of life, adversity is an inevitable thread, weaving its way through the fabric of our existence with unexpected twists and turns. Yet, amidst the storms of hardship and challenges, there exists a profound quality that empowers us to weather the tempests of life with grace and fortitude: resilience. Embracing resilience is not merely about enduring hardships; it's about harnessing the power within us to bounce back stronger, wiser, and more resilient than before. Here, we explore the essence of resilience and strategies to nurture this invaluable quality:

1. Understanding Resilience:

Resilience is more than just bouncing back; it's about adapting, growing, and thriving in the face of adversity. At its core, resilience is a dynamic process that encompasses emotional strength, mental flexibility, and a sense of purpose and meaning. It involves the ability to confront challenges with courage and optimism, recognizing setbacks as opportunities for growth and transformation.

2. Cultivating Self-Awareness:

The journey towards resilience begins with self-awareness—the ability to recognize and acknowledge our thoughts, emotions, and reactions to adversity. By cultivating mindfulness and introspection, we can gain insight into our inner strengths and limitations, allowing us to respond to challenges with greater clarity and resilience.

3. Building a Support Network:

No one is an island, and resilience thrives in the soil of supportive relationships. Surround yourself with friends, family, mentors, and peers who offer encouragement, guidance, and empathy during difficult times. Sharing your struggles with trusted confidants can provide perspective, validation, and a sense of connection that bolsters your resilience.

4. Practicing Adaptability:

Resilience is rooted in adaptability—the ability to pivot, innovate, and find creative solutions in the face of change and uncertainty. Embrace flexibility in your thinking and approach to challenges, reframing setbacks as opportunities for innovation and growth. Cultivate a mindset of curiosity and openness to new experiences, knowing that resilience thrives in the fertile soil of adaptability.

5. Developing Coping Strategies:

Resilience is not about avoiding stress or adversity but about developing effective coping strategies to navigate them. Identify healthy coping mechanisms that resonate with you, whether it's exercise, meditation, journaling, or spending time in nature. Cultivate self-care practices that nourish your body, mind, and soul, replenishing your reserves of resilience and fortitude.

6. Finding Meaning and Purpose:

Resilience is fuelled by a sense of meaning and purpose —a deep conviction that our struggles have significance and our lives have meaning. Reflect on your values, passions, and aspirations, and connect with a sense of purpose that transcends adversity. Find meaning in the lessons learned, the connections forged, and the growth experienced through life's challenges.

7. Embracing Growth Mindset:

Resilience thrives in the soil of a growth mindset—a belief that challenges are opportunities for learning and development. Cultivate a mindset of optimism and possibility, reframing setbacks as stepping stones on the path to success. Embrace a lifelong journey of growth and self-improvement, knowing that resilience is a muscle that strengthens with each trial overcome.

Embracing resilience is a journey of self-discovery and empowerment—a testament to the indomitable human spirit's capacity to overcome adversity and thrive in the face of challenges. By cultivating self-awareness, building a support network, practicing adaptability, developing coping strategies, finding meaning and purpose, and embracing a growth mindset, we can nurture the seeds of resilience within us and emerge from life's trials stronger, wiser, and more resilient than before. As we navigate the twists and turns of our journey, may we draw strength from the wellspring of resilience within us, knowing that every setback is but a stepping stone on the path to resilience and growth.

Chapter 3:

Cultivating a Positive Mindset

- Gratitude and Appreciation:

Embracing Gratitude as a Gateway to Positivity and Fulfilment.

- Mindfulness and Presence:

Practices to Anchor Oneself in the Present Moment and Savour Life's Joys.

- Self-Compassion:

Fostering Kindness and Acceptance Towards Oneself Amidst Life's Challenges.

Cultivating a Positive Mindset

In the garden of life, our mindset is the fertile soil from which our experiences grow. Just as a gardener tends to their plants with care and attention, so too must we nurture our minds to cultivate positivity and resilience. In a world often filled with challenges and uncertainties, fostering a positive mindset becomes not just a choice but a necessity for our well-being and success.

1. Cultivating Awareness

The first step in cultivating a positive mindset is to become aware of our thoughts and attitudes. Just as a gardener must assess the condition of their soil before planting, we must examine our mental landscape. Are our thoughts predominantly negative or positive? Do we tend to focus on our strengths or weaknesses? Awareness is the cornerstone upon which we can build a more positive outlook.

2. Planting Seeds of Positivity

Once we are aware of our thought patterns, we can begin to plant seeds of positivity. This involves deliberately choosing to focus on the good in ourselves, others, and the world around us. Like planting seeds in a garden, it requires patience and consistency. We can start small, acknowledging even the smallest victories and expressing gratitude for the blessings in our lives. Over time, these seeds of positivity will take root and flourish, transforming our mindset.

3. Nourishing Growth Through Self-Compassion

Just as plants need water and sunlight to thrive, our minds require nourishment in the form of self-compassion. Too often, we are our harshest critics, dwelling on our mistakes and shortcomings. Cultivating a positive mindset means treating ourselves with the same kindness and understanding that we would offer to a friend. Instead of berating ourselves for our imperfections, we can recognise them as opportunities for growth and learning

4. Embracing Challenges as Opportunities

In the garden of life, challenges are inevitable. However, rather than seeing them as obstacles, we can choose to view them as opportunities for growth. Just as plants grow stronger when subjected to adversity, so too can we develop resilience in the face of challenges. By reframing setbacks as opportunities for learning and development, we can cultivate a mindset that is not only positive but also resilient.

5. Cultivating Community and Connection

Just as plants thrive in a supportive ecosystem, so too do we flourish when surrounded by a positive and supportive community. Cultivating connections with others who uplift and inspire us can fuel our own positivity. Whether through friendships, mentorships, or support groups, these connections remind us that we are not alone in our journey. Together, we can cultivate a collective mindset of positivity and resilience.

Cultivating a positive mindset is not a one-time endeavour but an ongoing practice that requires patience, intention, and perseverance. Like tending to a garden, it requires attention to the seeds we plant, the nourishment we provide, and the environment in which we grow. By cultivating awareness, planting seeds of positivity, nurturing ourselves with self-compassion, embracing challenges as opportunities, and cultivating connections with others, we can cultivate a mindset that not only sustains us but allows us to thrive in the ever-changing landscape of life.

Gratitude and Appreciation:

Embracing Gratitude as a Gateway to Positivity and Fulfilment

In the tapestry of life, gratitude and appreciation weave threads of joy, contentment, and fulfilment. They are the gentle reminders that amidst life's chaos and challenges, there is always something to be thankful for. Embracing gratitude not only shifts our perspective but also serves as a gateway to a more positive and fulfilling existence.

1. The Power of Gratitude

Gratitude is more than just saying "thank you"; it is a profound acknowledgment of the blessings and abundance present in our lives. When we cultivate an attitude of gratitude, we train our minds to focus on the positive aspects of our experiences, no matter how small or seemingly insignificant. This shift in perspective has the power to transform even the darkest moments into opportunities for growth and appreciation.

2. Finding Beauty in the Ordinary

In a world that often glorifies grand achievements and material wealth, gratitude invites us to find beauty in the ordinary. From the warmth of the morning sun to the laughter of loved ones, there is magic to be found in the simplest of moments. By pausing to appreciate these everyday miracles, we cultivate a sense of wonder and awe that enriches our lives immeasurably.

3. Embracing Abundance Over Scarcity

In a culture of consumerism and comparison, it is easy to fall into the trap of scarcity thinking—the belief that there is never "enough" to go around. However, gratitude reminds us that abundance is not measured by material possessions but by the richness of our experiences and relationships. When we shift our focus from what we lack to what we have, we open ourselves up to a world of abundance and possibility.

4. Cultivating Resilience Through Gratitude

Gratitude is not just a tool for enhancing our mood; it is also a powerful resilience-building practice. When faced with adversity, acknowledging the things we are grateful for can provide a beacon of light in the darkness. It reminds us of our inner strength and resilience, empowering us to navigate life's challenges with grace and courage.

5. Spreading Positivity Through Appreciation

Just as a single candle can light up a dark room, so too can gratitude illuminate the lives of those around us. By expressing appreciation for others and their contributions, we not only uplift their spirits but also cultivate a culture of kindness and positivity. Whether through a heartfelt thank-you note or a simple act of kindness, we have the power to spread joy and goodwill wherever we go.

Gratitude and appreciation are not fleeting emotions but transformative practices that have the power to enrich our lives in profound ways. By embracing gratitude as a way of being, we unlock the door to positivity, fulfilment, and resilience. May we cultivate a heart overflowing with gratitude, sowing seeds of joy and abundance wherever we go.

Mindfulness and Presence:

Practices to Anchor Oneself in the Present Moment and Savour Life's Joys

In a world constantly buzzing with activity and distraction, the art of mindfulness and presence offers a sanctuary—a refuge where we can anchor ourselves in the present moment and savour life's joys. It is a practice that invites us to slow down, to breathe, and to fully engage with the richness of each moment, regardless of its simplicity or complexity. In the embrace of mindfulness, we discover that true fulfilment and contentment lie not in the past or future but in the here and now.

1. The Essence of Mindfulness

At its core, mindfulness is the practice of paying attention to the present moment with openness, curiosity, and acceptance. It is about cultivating a non-judgmental awareness of our thoughts, emotions, and sensations as they arise, without getting caught up in the stories they tell or the judgments they carry. In essence, mindfulness is the art of being fully alive, awake, and attuned to the unfolding of life as it happens.

2. Cultivating Presence Through Breath

One of the simplest and most powerful ways to cultivate mindfulness is through the breath. The breath serves as an anchor—a tether that connects us to the present moment amidst the ebb and flow of our thoughts and emotions. By bringing our attention to the sensations of the breath—its rise and fall, its warmth and coolness— we ground ourselves in the here and now, moment by moment.

3. Savouring Life's Joys

In the rush of everyday life, it is easy to overlook the simple pleasures that abound around us—the warmth of the sun on our skin, the laughter of a child, the aroma of freshly brewed coffee. Mindfulness invites us to slow down and savour these moments of joy and beauty, like a connoisseur relishing the subtle nuances of a fine wine. By fully immersing ourselves in the richness of each experience, we awaken to the beauty and wonder of life's tapestry.

4. Embracing Impermanence with Grace

Central to the practice of mindfulness is the recognition of impermanence—the understanding that all things, both pleasant and unpleasant, are transient and ever-changing. Rather than clinging to the past or grasping for an uncertain future, mindfulness teaches us to embrace each moment with grace and equanimity, knowing that it too shall pass. In doing so, we cultivate a deep sense of peace and acceptance that transcends the fluctuations of life.

5. Navigating Challenges with Resilience

Mindfulness is not just about savouring life's joys; it is also about navigating its challenges with resilience and grace. By cultivating a present-moment awareness of our thoughts, emotions, and bodily sensations, we develop the capacity to respond skilfully to difficult situations rather than reacting impulsively out of fear or aversion. In this way, mindfulness becomes a steadfast companion

—a source of strength and wisdom in the face of adversity.

In the sanctuary of mindfulness and presence, we discover a profound sense of aliveness—a deep-rooted connection to ourselves, to others, and to the world around us. It is a practice that invites us to awaken from the trance of busyness and distraction and to fully inhabit the precious moments of our lives. May we cultivate mindfulness with patience and perseverance, savouring each breath, each sensation, and each moment with an open heart and a spirit of wonder.

Self-Compassion:

Fostering Kindness and Acceptance Towards Oneself Amidst Life's Challenges

In the labyrinth of life's challenges and uncertainties, self-compassion emerges as a guiding light—a gentle reminder to treat ourselves with the same kindness and acceptance that we offer to others. It is a practice of cultivating warmth and understanding towards ourselves, even in the midst of our struggles and imperfections. In the embrace of self-compassion, we find solace, strength, and a profound sense of wholeness amidst life's inevitable difficulties.

1. The Heart of Self-Compassion

At its core, self-compassion is the practice of extending kindness, understanding, and acceptance to ourselves, especially in times of difficulty or suffering. It involves recognizing our own humanity—the fact that we are all imperfect beings navigating the complexities of life—and responding with a tender-heartedness that soothes and nurtures our spirit. Self-compassion is not about self-indulgence or self-pity but about holding ourselves with the same care and compassion that we would offer to a dear friend in need.

2. Embracing Imperfection with Grace

In a culture that often glorifies perfection and achievement, self-compassion offers a sanctuary—a safe haven where we can embrace our imperfections with grace and acceptance. Rather than berating ourselves for our mistakes or shortcomings, self-compassion invites us to recognize our inherent worthiness, regardless of our perceived flaws. It is an affirmation of our shared humanity—a recognition that imperfection is not a sign of weakness but a testament to our resilience and capacity for growth.

3. Cultivating a Nurturing Inner Dialogue

Central to the practice of self-compassion is the cultivation of a nurturing inner dialogue—a gentle and supportive voice that offers comfort and encouragement in times of need. Instead of harsh self-criticism or negative self-talk, self-compassion encourages us to speak to ourselves with kindness and understanding, as we would to a cherished friend. This shift in self-talk can be transformative, fostering a sense of inner peace and self-assurance that radiates outwards into every aspect of our lives.

4. Finding Strength in Vulnerability

Contrary to popular belief, self-compassion is not a sign of weakness but a source of profound strength and resilience. It takes courage to acknowledge our vulnerabilities and struggles—to sit with them, rather than push them away or suppress them. Yet, in the embrace of self-compassion, we discover that our vulnerabilities are not weaknesses to be hidden but badges of courage to be celebrated. They are a testament to our humanity and our capacity for empathy, connection, and growth.

5. Embracing Self-Care as an Act of Kindness

Self-compassion also encompasses the practice of self-care—an intentional commitment to nourishing our physical, emotional, and spiritual well-being. Just as we would care for a beloved garden, tending to its needs with love and attention, so too must we care for ourselves with the same tenderness and devotion. Whether through rest, relaxation, creative expression, or seeking support from others, self-care is an act of kindness—an affirmation of our inherent worthiness and value.

In the gentle embrace of self-compassion, we discover a reservoir of kindness, acceptance, and strength that sustains us through life's trials and tribulations. It is a practice that invites us to extend the same warmth and understanding to ourselves that we so readily offer to others. May we cultivate self-compassion with patience and gentleness, nurturing the tender seed of kindness within our hearts and minds, and embracing ourselves with love and acceptance on every step of life's journey.

Chapter 4:

Empowering Relationships

- The Power of Connection:

Exploring How Positive Relationships Enrich Our Lives and Nurture Our Well-being.

- Communicating with Positivity:

Techniques for Fostering Constructive Communication and Resolving Conflicts.

- Building Support Networks:

Cultivating Relationships That Uplift, Inspire, and Sustain us Through Life's Trials.

The Power of Connection:

Exploring How Positive Relationships Enrich Our Lives and Nurture Our Well-being

In the intricate tapestry of human existence, connections form the threads that weave together the fabric of our lives. From the fleeting encounters with strangers to the profound bonds shared with loved ones, these connections shape our experiences and influence our well-being in profound ways. In exploring the dynamics of human relationships, we uncover the transformative power of connection and its profound impact on our emotional, mental, and physical health.

At the heart of the human experience lies a fundamental longing for connection. We are inherently social beings, wired to seek out companionship, understanding, and support. From the moment we are born, we crave the warmth of human touch and the reassurance of belonging to a community. As we navigate through life's journey, these connections serve as beacons of light, guiding us through the darkest of times and amplifying the joy in moments of celebration.

Positive relationships act as catalysts for personal growth and fulfilment. When we forge meaningful connections with others, we create a fertile ground for empathy, compassion, and understanding to flourish. Through shared experiences and mutual support, we gain valuable insights into ourselves and the world around us, fostering a sense of belonging and acceptance.

Moreover, the benefits of positive relationships extend far beyond mere emotional satisfaction. Research has shown that nurturing strong social connections is closely linked to improved mental health and overall well-being. When we feel connected to others, our stress levels decrease, our immune systems strengthen, and our resilience in the face of adversity grows. In essence, the presence of supportive relationships acts as a buffer against life's inevitable challenges, providing us with the courage and fortitude to persevere.

Furthermore, the power of connection extends beyond individual well-being to encompass the broader fabric of society. When communities are built on a foundation of trust, cooperation, and mutual respect, they become resilient and vibrant ecosystems where individuals can thrive. Through acts of kindness, generosity, and solidarity, we create ripple effects that transcend boundaries, uniting us in our shared humanity.

In today's fast-paced world, where digital screens often replace face-to-face interactions and superficial connections abound, the importance of cultivating genuine relationships cannot be overstated. It is through meaningful conversations, heartfelt gestures, and moments of genuine connection that we truly enrich our lives and nurture our well-being.

As we navigate the complexities of modern life, let us remember the profound impact that positive relationships can have on our lives. Let us prioritize the cultivation of connections that uplift and inspire us and let us approach each interaction with an open heart and a willingness to connect deeply with others. For it is through the power of connection that we find meaning, purpose, and fulfilment in our shared journey through life.

Building Support Networks:

Cultivating Relationships That Uplift, Inspire, and sustain Us Through Life's Trials

In the tapestry of life, we encounter moments of joy, triumph, and fulfilment, but we also face challenges, setbacks, and uncertainties. It is during these times of trial that the importance of support networks becomes abundantly clear. Cultivating relationships that uplift, inspire, and sustain us is not only essential for navigating life's complexities but also for fostering resilience and growth in the face of adversity.

At the heart of a robust support network lies the foundation of trust and reciprocity. These relationships are characterized by mutual understanding, empathy, and a willingness to offer both emotional and practical support when needed. Whether it's a shoulder to lean on during times of sorrow, a listening ear to share our hopes and fears, or a helping hand to lighten our burdens, these connections serve as pillars of strength upon which we can lean.

Building a support network begins with the cultivation of authentic connections rooted in vulnerability and trust. By opening ourselves up to others and sharing our authentic selves, we create spaces for genuine rapport to develop. Whether it's through shared experiences, common interests, or a shared sense of purpose, these bonds deepen over time, offering a sense of belonging and acceptance that nourishes the soul.

Moreover, a diverse support network encompasses a variety of relationships that fulfil different needs and roles in our lives. From close friends and family members to mentors, colleagues, and members of our community, each connection brings a unique perspective and set of resources to the table. By diversifying our support network, we ensure that we have access to a broad range of perspectives, expertise, and support systems to draw upon in times of need.

In addition to offering emotional support, a strong support network can also serve as a source of inspiration and encouragement. Surrounding ourselves with individuals who believe in our potential and champion our dreams can fuel our motivation and propel us forward on our path to growth and self-discovery. Whether it's through words of affirmation, constructive feedback, or acts of encouragement, these relationships provide the encouragement and validation we need to pursue our goals with confidence and determination.

Furthermore, the reciprocal nature of support networks fosters a sense of interconnectedness and collective well-being. Just as we rely on others for support, we also have the opportunity to pay it forward and offer our own support to those in need. Through acts of kindness, generosity, and compassion, we strengthen the bonds of reciprocity within our communities, creating a ripple effect of positive change that extends far beyond ourselves.

In today's fast-paced world, where isolation and loneliness are all too common, the importance of building support networks cannot be overstated. By investing in meaningful relationships that uplift, inspire, and sustain us, we cultivate the resilience and inner strength needed to navigate life's challenges with grace and dignity.

As we journey through life's ups and downs, let us remember the transformative power of support networks. Let us nurture the connections that lift our spirits, bolster our courage, and remind us that we are never alone. For it is through the bonds of friendship, love, and community that we find solace, strength, and belonging on our shared journey through life.

Communicating with Positivity:

Techniques for Fostering Constructive Communication and Resolving Conflicts

In the tapestry of human interaction, communication serves as the vibrant thread that weaves together the fabric of relationships. At its core, communication is more than mere words exchanged; it is a dynamic interplay of thoughts, emotions, and intentions. In fostering positive communication, we unlock the potential for constructive dialogue, mutual understanding, and the resolution of conflicts.

Central to the art of positive communication is the cultivation of empathy and active listening. Too often, we approach conversations with the intent to speak rather than to truly understand. By practicing empathetic listening, we step into the shoes of others, seeking to comprehend their perspectives, feelings, and underlying needs. Through attentive listening and genuine curiosity, we create a safe space for open dialogue and the exchange of ideas.

Moreover, the language we choose shapes the tone and direction of our interactions. Embracing positivity in communication entails the mindful selection of words that uplift, inspire, and affirm. Rather than resorting to blame or criticism, we strive to express ourselves with kindness, respect, and authenticity. By framing our messages in a positive light, we foster an atmosphere of trust and collaboration, paving the way for productive discourse and conflict resolution.

In the face of conflict, positive communication offers a pathway to reconciliation and mutual growth. Rather than escalating tensions through defensiveness or aggression, we approach disagreements with a spirit of openness and flexibility. Through active listening, validation of feelings, and the use of "I" statements to express our own perspectives and emotions, we create a foundation for constructive dialogue. By reframing conflicts as opportunities for learning and understanding, we can work together to find mutually beneficial solutions that honour the needs and concerns of all parties involved.

Furthermore, nonverbal cues play a significant role in communication, often conveying messages more powerfully than words alone. Through attentive body language, such as maintaining eye contact, nodding in acknowledgment, and offering affirming gestures, we signal our engagement and receptivity to others. By aligning our verbal and nonverbal communication, we enhance the clarity and effectiveness of our message, fostering deeper connections and rapport.

In today's interconnected world, where misunderstandings can easily arise and conflicts abound, the practice of positive communication is more essential than ever. By embracing empathy, mindfulness, and authenticity in our interactions, we create spaces where understanding can flourish, and conflicts can be resolved with grace and dignity.

As we navigate the complexities of human relationships, let us remember the transformative power of positive communication. Let us approach each interaction with an open heart and a commitment to fostering connection, understanding, and mutual respect. For it is through the art of positive communication that we build bridges, mend divides, and cultivate a more harmonious world.

Chapter 5:

Pursuing Purpose and Meaning

- Aligning with Values:

Discovering and Living in Alignment with Personal Values and Aspirations.

- Finding Flow:

Engaging in Activities That Foster Immersion, Creativity, and a Sense of Purpose.

- Contribution and Service:

Harnessing the Transformative Power of Giving Back to Others and Making a Difference in the World.

Pursuing Purpose and Meaning

In the grand tapestry of existence, the quest for purpose and meaning serves as the guiding thread that weaves together the fabric of our lives. Rooted in the depths of our being, this innate longing propels us forward on a journey of self-discovery, growth, and fulfilment. Embracing positivity in this pursuit not only illuminates our path but also infuses our lives with a sense of joy, resilience, and purposeful living.

At the heart of pursuing purpose and meaning lies a deep-seated desire to align our actions with our values, passions, and aspirations. It is a journey of introspection and self-exploration, wherein we unearth the unique gifts, talents, and strengths that define us. By cultivating self-awareness and authenticity, we empower ourselves to live in alignment with our true selves, unleashing our full potential and embracing the richness of our individuality.

Embracing positivity in the pursuit of purpose and meaning entails adopting a mindset of gratitude, optimism, and possibility. Rather than dwelling on past regrets or future uncertainties, we focus our attention on the present moment, recognizing the abundance and beauty that surrounds us. Through a lens of positivity, even life's challenges become opportunities for growth, resilience, and transformation.

Moreover, positivity serves as a catalyst for resilience in the face of adversity. When we encounter obstacles or setbacks along our journey, maintaining a positive outlook enables us to navigate through them with grace and determination. Instead of succumbing to despair or defeat, we draw upon our inner strength and optimism to overcome obstacles, learn from setbacks, and emerge stronger and wiser than before.

In the pursuit of purpose and meaning, relationships play a vital role in amplifying our sense of fulfilment and connection. Surrounding ourselves with supportive, uplifting individuals who share our values and aspirations energizes us and inspires us to reach for the stars. Through collaboration, mutual encouragement, and acts of kindness, we cultivate a sense of belonging and community that enriches our lives and fuels our pursuit of purpose.

Furthermore, embracing positivity in the pursuit of purpose and meaning extends beyond individual fulfilment to encompass a broader sense of contribution and service to others. By aligning our actions with a greater sense of purpose that transcends our own self-interests, we become agents of positive change in the world. Whether it's through acts of kindness, advocacy for social justice, or creative expression, we make meaningful contributions that leave a lasting impact on the lives of others and the world around us.

In today's fast-paced world, where distractions abound and societal pressures often dictate our sense of worth and identity, the pursuit of purpose and meaning becomes more important than ever. By embracing positivity as our guiding light, we infuse our lives with a sense of joy, purpose, and meaning that transcends external circumstances and empowers us to live authentically and fully.

As we embark on this journey of self-discovery and growth, let us embrace positivity as our constant companion, illuminating our path and infusing our lives with meaning and purpose. For it is through the pursuit of purpose and meaning that we uncover the true essence of our being and realize our potential to create a life of significance and fulfilment.

Aligning with Values:

Discovering and Living in Alignment with Personal Values and Aspirations

In the labyrinth of life, the compass that guides us towards fulfilment and authenticity is our set of personal values. These intrinsic principles serve as the North Star, illuminating our path and shaping our choices, actions, and aspirations. Embracing positivity while aligning with our values is not only a transformative journey of self-discovery but also a pathway to living a life of purpose, meaning, and joy.

At the core of aligning with our values lies the process of self-discovery and introspection. It requires delving deep into the recesses of our hearts and minds, uncovering the beliefs, principles, and ideals that resonate most deeply with our authentic selves. By cultivating self-awareness and clarity about what truly matters to us, we pave the way for living in alignment with our values and aspirations.

Embracing positivity in this journey involves adopting a mindset of optimism, gratitude, and possibility. Rather than focusing on limitations or perceived shortcomings, we celebrate our strengths, talents, and unique qualities. Through a lens of positivity, we recognize the inherent potential within ourselves to live authentically and make meaningful contributions to the world around us.

Living in alignment with our values requires courage and commitment to honour our principles, even in the face of adversity or societal pressures. It entails making conscious choices that reflect our values and priorities, rather than succumbing to external expectations or influences. By staying true to ourselves and our convictions, we cultivate a sense of integrity and wholeness that empowers us to live with authenticity and purpose.

Moreover, aligning with our values fosters a sense of coherence and harmony in our lives. When our actions are congruent with our values, we experience a deep sense of inner peace and fulfilment. We no longer feel fragmented or conflicted, but rather grounded and centred in our sense of self. Through this alignment, we cultivate a profound sense of well-being that permeates every aspect of our lives.

Furthermore, living in alignment with our values enhances our relationships and connections with others. When we embody our values authentically, we attract like-minded individuals who share our principles and aspirations. Through meaningful connections and mutual support, we create a sense of belonging and community that enriches our lives and amplifies our collective impact on the world.

In today's fast-paced world, where external pressures and distractions abound, the importance of aligning with our values cannot be overstated. By embracing positivity as our guiding light, we embark on a transformative journey of self-discovery and growth. Through introspection, courage, and commitment, we align our lives with our deepest values and aspirations, creating a life of purpose, meaning, and joy.

As we navigate the complexities of life's journey, let us embrace positivity as our constant companion, illuminating our path and infusing our lives with authenticity and fulfilment. For it is through living in alignment with our values that we unlock the true essence of who we are and realize our potential to create a life of significance and impact.

Finding Flow:

Engaging in Activities That Foster immersion, Creativity, and a Sense of Purpose

In the rhythm of life, there exists a state of being where time seems to stand still, and every action flows effortlessly from one moment to the next. This is the state of flow—a transcendent experience characterized by deep immersion, heightened focus, and a profound sense of fulfilment. Engaging in activities that foster flow not only unleashes our creativity but also cultivates a profound sense of purpose and joy in our lives.

At the heart of finding flow lies the pursuit of activities that align with our passions, interests, and natural talents. Whether it's painting, writing, playing music, gardening, or solving complex problems, these activities captivate our attention and spark our curiosity, drawing us into a state of effortless concentration and absorption. By immersing ourselves in activities that resonate deeply with our souls, we tap into a wellspring of creativity and inspiration that fuels our sense of purpose and fulfilment.

Embracing positivity in the pursuit of flow involves adopting a mindset of openness, curiosity, and possibility. Rather than approaching activities with a sense of obligation or pressure to perform, we cultivate a sense of joy and wonder in the process itself. Through a lens of positivity, even challenges and setbacks become opportunities for growth and learning, enriching our experience and deepening our connection to the task at hand.

Moreover, finding flow fosters a sense of intrinsic motivation and autonomy in our lives. When we engage in activities that bring us joy and fulfilment, we are driven by an inner sense of purpose rather than external rewards or validation. This autonomy empowers us to explore our passions, take risks, and express ourselves authentically, leading to a deeper sense of satisfaction and meaning in our lives.

In the state of flow, time seems to dissolve, and we enter a state of effortless action where our skills and challenges are perfectly matched. This optimal balance between skill and challenge, known as the flow channel, allows us to experience a sense of mastery and accomplishment that transcends ego and self-doubt. In this state, we are fully present in the moment, completely absorbed in the task at hand, and free from the distractions of past regrets or future worries.

Furthermore, finding flow fosters a sense of interconnectedness and unity with the world around us. When we are immersed in activities that bring us joy and fulfilment, we feel deeply connected to ourselves, others, and the larger universe. Through our creative expression and engagement with the world, we contribute to a collective tapestry of beauty, meaning, and interconnectedness that enriches the human experience.

In today's fast-paced world, where distractions and demands abound, the pursuit of flow offers a sanctuary of peace, creativity, and purpose. By embracing positivity as our guiding light, we embark on a transformative journey of self-discovery and growth. Through immersion in activities that ignite our passions and spark our curiosity, we tap into a wellspring of creativity and inspiration that enriches our lives and uplifts the world around us.

As we navigate the complexities of life's journey, let us embrace the flow as our constant companion, guiding us towards deeper connection, creativity, and fulfilment. For it is through finding flow that we unlock the true essence of who we are and realize our potential to create a life of meaning, purpose, and joy.

Contribution and Service:

Harnessing the Transformative Power of Giving Back to Others and Making a Difference in the World

In the symphony of human existence, there exists a profound melody that resonates with the spirit of generosity, compassion, and altruism. It is the song of contribution and service—a call to action that beckons us to extend a helping hand, uplift those in need, and make a positive impact in the world. Harnessing the transformative power of giving back not only enriches the lives of others but also nourishes our own souls, fostering a sense of purpose, fulfilment, and interconnectedness.

At the heart of contribution and service lies the recognition of our shared humanity and interconnectedness. When we extend ourselves in service to others, we transcend the boundaries of self-interest and ego, forging bonds of compassion and empathy that unite us in our common humanity. Whether it's through acts of kindness, volunteerism, or advocacy for social justice, these gestures of generosity ripple outward, creating waves of positive change that reverberate throughout society.

Embracing positivity in the spirit of contribution and service involves cultivating a mindset of abundance, gratitude, and empathy. Rather than focusing on scarcity or limitations, we recognize the abundance of resources, talents, and opportunities at our disposal. Through a lens of positivity, we approach service as a privilege and an opportunity to express gratitude for the blessings in our own lives by uplifting others.

Moreover, giving back fosters a profound sense of purpose and meaning in our lives. When we align our actions with a greater sense of contribution and service, we tap into a wellspring of fulfilment that transcends personal gain or achievement. Whether it's mentoring a young person, supporting a cause we believe in, or lending a helping hand to a neighbour in need, these acts of service imbue our lives with a sense of significance and impact that resonates deeply with our souls.

In the act of giving, we also discover the transformative power of connection and community. When we come together in service to a shared cause or vision, we forge bonds of solidarity and unity that transcend individual differences and divisions. Through collaboration, mutual support, and collective action, we amplify our impact and create a ripple effect of positive change that extends far beyond our individual efforts.

Furthermore, giving back nurtures a sense of empowerment and agency in our lives. When we take action to address the needs and challenges facing our communities, we reclaim a sense of control and agency over our own destinies. Rather than passively accepting the status quo, we become agents of change, actively shaping a future that reflects our values, aspirations, and vision for a more just and compassionate world.

In today's complex and interconnected world, where divisiveness and discord often dominate the headlines, the importance of contribution and service cannot be overstated. By embracing positivity as our guiding light, we embark on a transformative journey of self-discovery and growth. Through acts of generosity, compassion, and service, we not only make a difference in the lives of others but also nurture our own souls, fostering a sense of purpose, fulfilment, and interconnectedness that enriches the human experience.

As we navigate the complexities of life's journey, let us heed the call to contribution and service, embracing the transformative power of giving back and making a positive impact in the world. For it is through acts of kindness, compassion, and generosity that we unlock the true potential of our humanity and create a brighter, more compassionate world for all.

Chapter 6:

Navigating Challenges with Optimism

- Resilient Optimism:

Cultivating a Resilient Mindset That Sees Setbacks as Opportunities for Growth.

- Adaptive Coping Strategies:

Techniques for Navigating Challenges with Grace, Creativity, and Resilience.

- The Role of Perspective:

Harnessing the Power of Perspective to Find Meaning and Wisdom in Life's Trials.

Challenges with Optimism

Life is a journey marked by peaks and valleys, where challenges and obstacles often punctuate the path, we tread. In the face of adversity, the transformative power of optimism shines as a beacon of hope, guiding us through the darkest of times and illuminating the way forward. Embracing positivity while navigating challenges not only strengthens our resilience but also empowers us to find meaning, growth, and opportunity amidst the trials we encounter.

At the heart of navigating challenges with optimism lies the choice to see setbacks as opportunities for growth and learning. Instead of succumbing to despair or defeat, we adopt a mindset of resilience and resourcefulness, viewing obstacles as stepping stones rather than stumbling blocks. Through a lens of positivity, even the most daunting challenges become catalysts for personal transformation and self-discovery.

Embracing positivity in the face of adversity involves cultivating a sense of hope, courage, and determination.

Rather than dwelling on limitations or past failures, we focus our attention on possibilities and solutions. By maintaining a hopeful outlook and belief in our ability to overcome obstacles, we tap into an inner reservoir of strength and resilience that empowers us to persevere in the face of adversity.

Moreover, navigating challenges with optimism fosters a sense of empowerment and agency in our lives. When we approach difficulties with a positive mindset, we reclaim control over our narrative and become active participants in shaping our own destinies. Rather than allowing circumstances to dictate our sense of worth or identity, we draw upon our inner resources and creativity to chart a course towards a brighter future.

In the midst of adversity, we also discover the transformative power of connection and support. When we reach out to others for encouragement, guidance, or a listening ear, we forge bonds of solidarity and compassion that sustain us through the storm. Through acts of kindness, empathy, and mutual support, we create a network of support that reminds us we are never alone in our struggles.

Furthermore, navigating challenges with optimism fosters a sense of gratitude and appreciation for the blessings in our lives. Even in the midst of adversity, we find moments of beauty, kindness, and grace that remind us of the inherent goodness in the world. By cultivating an attitude of gratitude, we shift our focus from what is lacking to what is abundant, finding solace and strength in the simple joys that surround us.

In today's uncertain and volatile world, where challenges abound and uncertainties loom large, the importance of navigating adversity with optimism cannot be overstated. By embracing positivity as our guiding light, we embark on a transformative journey of self-discovery and growth. Through resilience, hope, and courage, we navigate the challenges that lie before us, emerging stronger, wiser, and more compassionate than before.

As we navigate the peaks and valleys of life's journey, let us heed the call to navigate challenges with optimism, embracing the transformative power of positivity in the face of adversity. For it is through optimism that we find the strength to persevere, the courage to overcome, and the resilience to thrive, even in the darkest of times.

Resilient Optimism:

Cultivating a Resilient Mindset That Sees Setbacks as Opportunities for Growth

Setbacks and challenges are inevitable threads woven into the fabric of our journey. Yet, it is the resilient optimist who possesses the remarkable ability to transform adversity into opportunity, seeing setbacks not as stumbling blocks, but as stepping stones to personal growth and fulfilment. Cultivating a mindset of resilient optimism empowers us to navigate life's twists and turns with grace, courage, and resilience, ultimately leading to greater positivity and well-being.

At the heart of resilient optimism lies the belief that setbacks are not permanent roadblocks but temporary detours on the path to success. Instead of viewing challenges as insurmountable obstacles, the resilient optimist sees them as opportunities for learning, adaptation, and growth. By reframing setbacks as valuable lessons and opportunities for self-discovery, we unlock the potential for personal transformation and resilience in the face of adversity.

Embracing resilient optimism involves cultivating a mindset of flexibility, adaptability, and perseverance. Rather than dwelling on past failures or dwelling on the negatives, we focus our energy on finding solutions, exploring new possibilities, and moving forward with confidence and determination. Through resilience, we develop the inner strength and courage to confront challenges head-on, knowing that every setback is an opportunity for growth and development.

Moreover, resilient optimism fosters a sense of empowerment and agency in our lives. When we approach setbacks with a positive outlook, we reclaim control over our narratives and become active participants in shaping our destinies. Instead of allowing circumstances to dictate our sense of worth or identity, we draw upon our inner resources and creativity to chart a course towards a brighter future, filled with possibility and potential.

In the face of adversity, resilient optimism also fosters a sense of connection and support. When we reach out to others for encouragement, guidance, or a listening ear, we forge bonds of solidarity and compassion that sustain us through the storm. Through acts of kindness, empathy, and mutual support, we create a network of support that reminds us we are never alone in our struggles.

Furthermore, resilient optimism cultivates a sense of gratitude and appreciation for the blessings in our lives. Even in the midst of adversity, we find moments of beauty, kindness, and grace that remind us of the inherent goodness in the world. By cultivating an attitude of gratitude, we shift our focus from what is lacking to what is abundant, finding solace and strength in the simple joys that surround us.

In today's uncertain and challenging world, the importance of cultivating resilient optimism cannot be overstated. By embracing resilience and optimism as guiding principles, we empower ourselves to navigate life's ups and downs with courage, grace, and resilience. Through resilience, optimism, and a belief in our own ability to overcome adversity, we cultivate a mindset that sees setbacks not as roadblocks, but as opportunities for growth and transformation in positivity.

Adaptive Coping Strategies:

Techniques for Navigating Challenges with Grace, Creativity, and Resilience

Life is a journey filled with ups and downs, twists and turns, and unexpected challenges that test our resilience and fortitude. In the face of adversity, the ability to adapt and cope effectively is essential for maintaining a sense of balance, well-being, and positivity. By embracing adaptive coping strategies, we empower ourselves to navigate life's challenges with grace, creativity, and resilience, ultimately emerging stronger and more resilient in the process.

At the core of adaptive coping strategies lies the recognition that change is inevitable and that we possess the inner resources to navigate it with resilience and grace. Rather than resisting or avoiding challenges, we approach them with an open mind and a willingness to learn and grow. By embracing flexibility and adaptability, we harness the power to transform obstacles into opportunities for personal growth and development.

Embracing adaptive coping strategies involves cultivating a mindset of optimism, creativity, and resourcefulness. Instead of succumbing to despair or defeat in the face of adversity, we tap into our innate strengths and talents to find innovative solutions and pathways forward. By reframing setbacks as temporary hurdles on the road to success, we empower ourselves to overcome obstacles with resilience and determination.

Moreover, adaptive coping strategies foster a sense of empowerment and agency in our lives. When we approach challenges with a proactive mindset, we reclaim control over our narratives and become active participants in shaping our destinies. Rather than allowing circumstances to dictate our sense of worth or identity, we draw upon our inner resources and creativity to chart a course towards a brighter future, filled with possibility and potential.

In the face of adversity, adaptive coping strategies also foster a sense of connection and support. When we reach out to others for encouragement, guidance, or a listening ear, we forge bonds of solidarity and compassion that sustain us through the storm. Through acts of kindness, empathy, and mutual support, we create a network of support that reminds us we are never alone in our struggles.

Furthermore, adaptive coping strategies cultivate a sense of resilience and well-being that enables us to thrive in the face of uncertainty and change. By embracing resilience as a guiding principle, we develop the inner strength and courage to confront challenges head-on, knowing that every setback is an opportunity for growth and development. Through resilience, optimism, and a belief in our own ability to overcome adversity, we cultivate a mindset that sees challenges not as roadblocks, but as opportunities for growth and transformation.

The importance of adaptive coping strategies cannot be overstated. By embracing flexibility, creativity, and resilience as guiding principles, we empower ourselves to navigate life's challenges with grace, creativity, and resilience. Through adaptive coping strategies, we cultivate the resilience and fortitude needed to thrive in the face of adversity, emerging stronger, wiser, and more resilient in the process.

The Role of Perspective:

Harnessing the Power of Perspective to Find Meaning and Wisdom in Life's Trials

The lens through which we view the world shapes our perceptions, interpretations, and responses to life's trials and tribulations. The role of perspective cannot be overstated, for it holds the transformative power to shift our focus from adversity to opportunity, from despair to resilience, and from challenges to growth. By harnessing the power of perspective with positivity, we unlock the potential to find meaning, wisdom, and grace in even the darkest of times.

At the heart of harnessing the power of perspective lies the recognition that our interpretations of events are not fixed truths, but subjective constructs shaped by our beliefs, values, and experiences. Rather than viewing challenges as insurmountable obstacles, we cultivate a mindset that sees them as opportunities for growth, learning, and self-discovery. By reframing setbacks as temporary detours on the journey of life, we empower ourselves to transcend adversity and emerge stronger and more resilient in the process.

Embracing positivity in the face of adversity involves cultivating a sense of gratitude, resilience, and optimism. Instead of dwelling on the negatives or focusing solely on what is lacking, we shift our attention to the blessings, opportunities, and lessons that abound in every situation. Through a lens of positivity, even the most difficult circumstances become catalysts for personal growth, transformation, and empowerment.

Moreover, harnessing the power of perspective fosters a sense of agency and empowerment in our lives. When we recognize that we have the power to choose how we interpret and respond to life's challenges, we reclaim control over our narratives and become active participants in shaping our destinies. Rather than allowing circumstances to dictate our sense of worth or identity, we draw upon our inner resources and creativity to navigate adversity with grace and resilience.

In the face of adversity, perspective also plays a crucial role in fostering resilience and well-being. When we adopt a growth-oriented mindset that sees setbacks as opportunities for learning and development, we cultivate the inner strength and courage to confront challenges head-on. Through resilience, optimism, and a belief in our own ability to overcome adversity, we cultivate a mindset that sees challenges not as roadblocks, but as stepping stones to personal growth and transformation.

Furthermore, harnessing the power of perspective fosters a sense of connection and compassion for others. When we recognize that everyone experiences trials and tribulations in life, we develop empathy and understanding for the struggles of others. Through acts of kindness, empathy, and mutual support, we create a network of support that reminds us we are never alone in our struggles.

The importance of harnessing the power of perspective cannot be overstated. By embracing positivity as our guiding light, we empower ourselves to navigate life's challenges with grace, resilience, and wisdom. Through perspective, we cultivate the resilience and fortitude needed to thrive in the face of adversity, emerging stronger, wiser, and more compassionate in the process.

Chapter 7:

Sustaining Positivity Amidst Adversity

- Weathering Storms:

 Strategies for Maintaining Positivity during Times of Crisis, Uncertainty, and Grief.

- The Role of Self-Care:

Prioritising Self-care Practices that Nourish the Mind, Body, and Spirit.

- Seeking Support:

Leveraging the Support of Others and Seeking Professional Help When Needed.

Sustaining Positivity Amidst Adversity

Life's journey is often marked by unforeseen challenges and trials that can test our resolve and shake our sense of optimism. In the midst of adversity, sustaining positivity becomes a beacon of light guiding us through the darkest of times. Nurturing resilience amidst adversity involves cultivating a mindset of strength, hope, and perseverance that empowers us to navigate life's storms with grace and courage.

At the core of sustaining positivity amidst adversity lies the recognition that our outlook is a choice—a conscious decision to focus on the light even when surrounded by darkness. It's acknowledging the difficulties we face while also embracing the belief that we have the inner strength and resources to overcome them. By cultivating resilience, we shift our perspective from seeing challenges as insurmountable obstacles to viewing them as opportunities for growth and learning.

Embracing positivity amidst adversity involves nurturing a sense of gratitude, optimism, and hope. Instead of dwelling on the negatives or succumbing to despair, we train our minds to seek out the silver linings and blessings hidden within the storm. Through a lens of positivity, even the most difficult circumstances become opportunities for personal growth, resilience, and transformation.

Moreover, sustaining positivity amidst adversity requires practicing self-care and compassion towards oneself. It's about recognizing our limitations and giving ourselves permission to rest, recharge, and seek support when needed. By prioritizing our well-being and nurturing a sense of self-compassion, we build the resilience needed to weather life's storms with grace and dignity.

In the face of adversity, sustaining positivity also involves seeking support and connection with others. It's about reaching out to friends, family, or professional support networks for guidance, encouragement, and understanding. Through acts of kindness, empathy, and mutual support, we create a network of resilience that reminds us we are never alone in our struggles.

Furthermore, sustaining positivity amidst adversity entails embracing a growth mindset that sees setbacks as opportunities for learning and development. Instead of viewing challenges as roadblocks, we approach them with curiosity and openness, knowing that they hold the potential to strengthen our resilience and expand our capacity for empathy and compassion.

The importance of sustaining positivity amidst adversity cannot be overstated. By embracing resilience as a guiding principle, we empower ourselves to navigate life's challenges with grace, courage, and dignity. Through sustained positivity, we cultivate the inner strength and fortitude needed to thrive in the face of adversity, emerging stronger, wiser, and more compassionate in the process.

Weathering Storms:

Strategies for Maintaining Positivity During Times of Crisis, Uncertainty, and Grief

Life's journey is often characterized by unexpected storms—moments of crisis, uncertainty, and grief that can leave us feeling overwhelmed and adrift. In the face of such challenges, maintaining positivity becomes not only a beacon of hope but also a lifeline guiding us through the darkness. Weathering storms requires resilience, courage, and an unwavering commitment to nurturing positivity amidst adversity.

At the core of weathering storms lies the recognition that while we may not always have control over external circumstances, we have the power to choose how we respond to them. It's about embracing a mindset of resilience and optimism that empowers us to find light in the midst of darkness, hope in the face of despair, and strength in times of weakness.

Embracing positivity amidst crisis, uncertainty, and grief involves acknowledging our feelings and emotions with compassion and acceptance. It's about allowing ourselves

to experience the full range of human emotions—
sadness, anger, fear, and grief—without judgment or self-
condemnation. By honouring our emotions and giving
ourselves permission to feel, we create space for healing
and growth amidst adversity.

Moreover, maintaining positivity amidst storms requires
cultivating a sense of gratitude, resilience, and hope. It's
about shifting our focus from what is lost to what
remains, from what we cannot control to what we can,
and from despair to possibility. Through a lens of
positivity, even the darkest of moments become
opportunities for resilience, growth, and transformation.

In the face of crisis, uncertainty, and grief, maintaining
positivity also entails practicing self-care and compassion
towards oneself. It's about prioritizing our well-being and
nurturing our physical, emotional, and spiritual health
amidst adversity. Whether it's through mindfulness,
meditation, exercise, or creative expression, self-care
serves as a vital lifeline that sustains us through life's
storms.

Furthermore, maintaining positivity amidst storms involves seeking support and connection with others. It's about reaching out to friends, family, or professional support networks for guidance, encouragement, and understanding. Through acts of kindness, empathy, and mutual support, we create a network of resilience that reminds us we are never alone in our struggles.

In times of crisis, uncertainty, and grief, maintaining positivity also entails embracing a growth mindset that sees challenges as opportunities for learning and development. It's about approaching adversity with curiosity and openness, knowing that it holds the potential to strengthen our resilience, deepen our empathy, and cultivate our capacity for compassion.

The importance of maintaining positivity amidst storms cannot be overstated. By embracing resilience as a guiding principle, we empower ourselves to navigate life's challenges with grace, courage, and dignity. Through sustained positivity, we cultivate the inner strength and fortitude needed to weather the storms of life, emerging stronger, wiser, and more compassionate in the process.

The Role of Self-Care: Prioritising self-care practices that nourish the mind, body, and spirit

In the hustle and bustle of modern life, amidst its demands and distractions, it's easy to overlook the importance of self-care. Yet, at its core, self-care is not a luxury but a necessity—a vital practice that nourishes the mind, body, and spirit, fostering a sense of well-being and positivity. Prioritizing self-care is an act of self-love and compassion that empowers us to navigate life's challenges with grace, resilience, and optimism.

At the heart of self-care lies the recognition that our well-being is a holistic endeavour, encompassing the health of our mind, body, and spirit. It's about nurturing ourselves on all levels—physically, emotionally, mentally, and spiritually—to cultivate a sense of balance, vitality, and inner peace. By prioritizing self-care practices, we honour our innate worth and value, affirming our right to nourish and replenish ourselves in a world that often demands our constant attention and energy.

Embracing self-care involves cultivating a mindset of self-compassion, acceptance, and forgiveness. It's about recognizing our inherent worthiness and deservingness of love and care, regardless of external achievements or expectations. By treating ourselves with kindness and gentleness, we create a foundation of self-love and resilience that enables us to weather life's storms with grace and dignity.

Moreover, self-care encompasses a diverse array of practices and activities that nurture our physical, emotional, and spiritual well-being. From mindfulness meditation and yoga to exercise, nutritious eating, and adequate sleep, self-care involves prioritizing activities that promote vitality, resilience, and longevity. By tending to our physical health, we lay the groundwork for emotional stability, mental clarity, and spiritual growth.

In addition to physical self-care, nurturing our emotional and mental well-being is equally important. This may involve setting boundaries, saying no to commitments that drain our energy, and cultivating healthy coping mechanisms for managing stress and anxiety. Through practices such as journaling, therapy, or engaging in creative expression, we create space to process our emotions, gain insight into our inner world, and cultivate a greater sense of self-awareness and emotional resilience.

Furthermore, self-care encompasses nurturing our spiritual well-being—the essence of our innermost being and connection to something greater than ourselves. This may involve spending time in nature, engaging in practices of prayer or meditation, or connecting with a supportive community that shares our values and beliefs. By nourishing our spiritual selves, we cultivate a sense of meaning, purpose, and interconnectedness that sustains us through life's ups and downs.

The importance of prioritizing self-care cannot be overstated. By embracing self-care as a non-negotiable

aspect of our daily lives, we empower ourselves to thrive
—not just survive—in the face of life's challenges.
Through self-care practices that nurture the mind, body,
and spirit, we cultivate a reservoir of positivity,
resilience, and well-being that enables us to live with
greater joy, vitality, and purpose.

Seeking Support: Leveraging the support of others and seeking professional help when needed.

In the journey of life, there are moments when the weight of challenges and setbacks can feel overwhelming, leaving us drained of positivity and hope. In these times, seeking support becomes not only a lifeline but a courageous act of self-care and empowerment. By leveraging the support of others and seeking professional help when needed, we open ourselves to a wealth of resources and guidance that can help us regain our sense of positivity and well-being.

At the heart of seeking support lies the recognition that we do not have to navigate life's challenges alone. Whether it's leaning on friends, family, or trusted mentors, reaching out for support is a courageous step towards reclaiming our sense of positivity and resilience. By sharing our struggles and vulnerabilities with others, we invite compassion, empathy, and understanding into our lives, creating a network of support that sustains us through difficult times.

Embracing support involves cultivating a mindset of openness, vulnerability, and trust. It's about recognizing that asking for help is not a sign of weakness but a courageous act of self-awareness and self-compassion. By acknowledging our need for support and reaching out to others, we create opportunities for connection, healing, and growth that can profoundly impact our journey towards reclaiming positivity.

Moreover, seeking support may also involve reaching out to professional help when needed. Whether it's therapy, counselling, or coaching, professional support offers a safe and confidential space to explore our thoughts, feelings, and experiences in depth. Through therapeutic interventions and evidence-based techniques, we can gain insight into our patterns of thinking and behaviour, develop coping strategies for managing stress and adversity, and cultivate a greater sense of self-awareness and empowerment.

In addition to individual support, group support can also be incredibly valuable in reclaiming positivity and resilience. Whether it's joining a support group, attending workshops or seminars, or participating in community events, group support offers a sense of belonging and camaraderie that can help us feel less alone in our struggles. By connecting with others who share similar experiences, we gain validation, encouragement, and inspiration to keep moving forward on our journey towards reclaiming positivity.

Furthermore, seeking support involves prioritizing self-compassion and self-care as we navigate the ups and downs of life. It's about recognizing our own worth and deservingness of love and care, and treating ourselves with kindness, gentleness, and patience. By prioritizing our well-being and nurturing our physical, emotional, and spiritual health, we create a solid foundation of resilience and positivity that enables us to weather life's storms with grace and courage.

In today's complex and demanding world, the importance of seeking support cannot be overstated. By embracing support as an essential aspect of our journey towards reclaiming positivity, we empower ourselves to thrive—not just survive—in the face of life's challenges. Whether it's through the support of friends, family, or professional help, seeking support offers a pathway to healing, growth, and resilience that can transform our lives in profound and meaningful ways.

Embracing Positivity:

A Call to Radiate Transformative Energy into the World

As we reflect on the power of positivity and its profound impact on our lives, we are reminded of the immense potential we hold to cultivate a brighter, more compassionate future for ourselves and for humanity as a whole. In the midst of life's challenges and uncertainties, embracing positivity becomes not only a personal choice but a revolutionary act—a beacon of hope that illuminates the path towards healing, growth, and transformation.

At the heart of embracing positivity lies the recognition that we have the power to shape our own reality through our thoughts, words, and actions. By choosing optimism over pessimism, kindness over cruelty, and love over fear, we tap into a wellspring of resilience and inner strength that empowers us to navigate life's challenges with grace and courage.

Moreover, embracing positivity invites us to become beacons of light in a world that often feels shrouded in darkness. By radiating positivity and compassion into the world, we inspire others to do the same, creating a ripple effect of kindness, empathy, and healing that reverberates far beyond our individual spheres of influence.

As we embark on our own journey towards cultivating positivity, let us heed the call to action and commit ourselves to the following:

1. Cultivate self-awareness: Take time to reflect on your thoughts, beliefs, and attitudes towards yourself and the world around you. Cultivate mindfulness practices that help you become more present and aware of the present moment.

2. Practice gratitude: Cultivate an attitude of gratitude by regularly reflecting on the blessings, opportunities, and moments of joy in your life. Keep a gratitude journal or simply take a moment each day to express gratitude for the small miracles that surround you.

3. Choose kindness: Look for opportunities to extend kindness, compassion, and empathy towards others, even in the face of adversity. Small acts of kindness can have a ripple effect, creating positive change in the world around us.

4. Seek support: Reach out to friends, family, or professional support networks when needed. Seeking support is a courageous act of self-care and empowerment that can help us navigate life's challenges with grace and resilience.

5. Be the change: Embody the values of positivity, compassion, and resilience in your daily life. Lead by example and inspire others to embrace positivity and kindness as guiding principles in their own lives.

By embracing positivity, we not only enhance our own lives but also contribute to the collective well-being of humanity. Together, let us illuminate the path towards a brighter, more compassionate future, one small act of kindness at a time. The journey begins within each of us, as we harness the transformative power of positivity to create a world filled with love, compassion, and possibility.